Table of contents

THE BOOT CAMPER

Photography credit for photos of the author.
GeorgeRabe.net | DavidGoodmanPhotography.net

Welcome

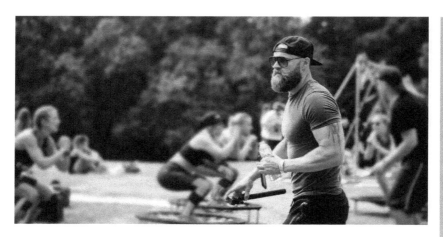

I wanted to start by thanking you for buying this book. Taking this time to discover how to lose the unwanted fat, tone up, get healthier and improve your lifestyle. This book will help you become the very best version of yourself.

I also want to congratulate you. This was more than likely a big step for you and I applaud you for taking the action needed to transform your body.

I remember when I started on my health and fitness journey, it was a big leap for me but learning how to transform my body was literally one of the best things I ever did. So well done, you won't regret it. Give yourself a pat on the back because this is going to be an absolute game changer for you! I know it, because I have done it.

Before we start I want to let you know that I am a qualified personal trainer and I genuinely practice what I preach. I am here to help you. I've got your back. I post regular tips and tricks to help you via my personal social media channels and I run a successful fitness boot camp in West Sussex, UK.

Follow me personally at:

BenHulme.com
Facebook.com/benhulmeofficial
Instagram.com/benhulme

Follow my boot camp at:

BootCampAtTulleys.com
Facebook.com/bootcampattulleys
Instagram.com/bootcampattulleys

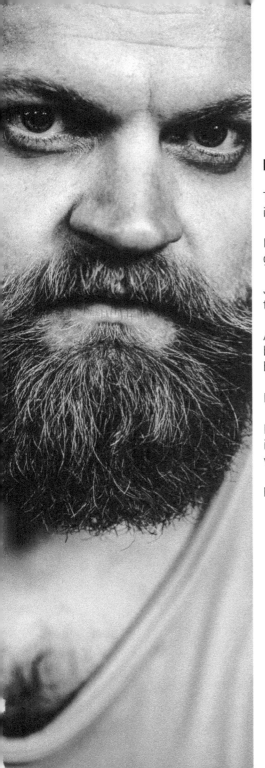

Life's Short. Live Well.

Thanks for being part of my journey to inspire a million people.

I will never be able to fully explain how grateful I am.

Just know that your support means the world to me.

All of this started from very humble beginnings, when all I wanted was to better myself for my daughters.

Now we are literally changing lives.

Never quit on your goals. Be relentless in your mission to become the best version of yourself.

Ben

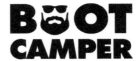

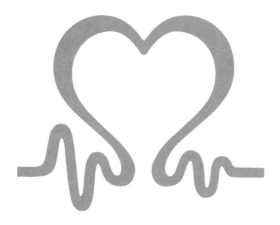

Beat Heartbreak Forever

IT STARTS WITH YOUR

Heart disease, stroke, vascular dementia
and diabetes are all connected.

That's why the British Heart Foundation
research starts with your heart, but doesn't stop there.

Visit **BHF.ORG.UK** to discover the amazing work they do.

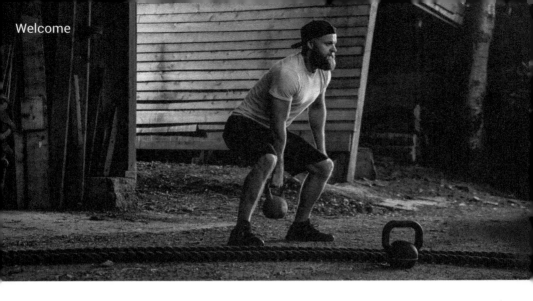

I live this life and I am proud to say that my clients have had amazing success stories, so I know just how powerful this nutrition plan can be – now it's your turn.

Yes, I am a qualified personal trainer but more importantly, I have been on my own personal journey. This means that I can personally train my boot campers and you with empathy as I know what a struggle it can be.

I used to be overweight and depressed, I have lived that life myself and I must say that being fit and healthy is so much better and I really hope that you fully commit to this to discover just how amazing you can feel!

I have fine tuned and followed this nutrition plan for many years and it has totally changed my life. You can literally change yours too. I am super excited for you to follow this nutrition plan and I can't wait for you to share your results with me.

I have learned so much during my transformation and even though I really hate the scales (more on this later) I just wanted to give you an idea of what I have achieved during my own journey.

In total I lost 5.7 stone (80lbs / 36kg) in 2 years and I have kept the fat off. I have gone on to build muscle and I am now, at the time of writing this, in the best shape of my life. I guarantee that if you stick to this and exercise regularly you will be amazed at what you can achieve.

When I started my body transformation journey I was not in a good place. I will share my story with you so you can see why helping other people is so close to my heart.

What you need to know is that nutrition is the secret to success with this, not just the exercise, it's what you eat that really makes the difference. It's important that you focus on your nutrition because exercise can only get you so far. It all comes down to the food and drink you consume and the lifestyle you live.

This is essentially what makes a body transformation successful, or not. Remember, it takes time. Be realistic, please! It frustrates me because I find that people have become accustomed to living in a society where we get what we want almost instantly.

They expect to see results in a couple of days but the reality is that our bodies were designed thousands of years ago. It takes time to adapt so don't rush this. Be patient and enjoy the process.

We are designed to adapt and change but over time, not instantly.

I always tell my boot campers:

- **4 weeks you will feel it**
- **8 weeks you will see it**
- **12 weeks you will hear it from others**

Remember to be realistic and take measurements to keep yourself accountable. By being realistic, your new healthy lifestyle will become sustainable. By taking on fad diets for a 'quick fix' you will put the fat back on and most likely more. Trust me, I have done that before!

I like to keep things really simple, thus making them sustainable. My belief is that it's what we consume when no one is watching that really makes this succeed to fail. This nutrition plan won't leave you craving the bad foods all the time, in fact you shouldn't really feel hungry ever! If you feel hungry then usually you are not eating enough.

I hope that this changes your life forever like it has mine. I am very excited to hear your results with this plan because I genuinely believe that this is the last nutrition plan you will ever need.

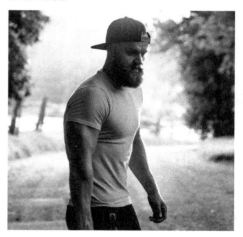

Disclaimer

**This guide cannot be sold or given away to anyone.
It is your personal copy only.**

Before you start you agree that:

None of what I am sharing with you here should damage your health in any way. However by using this information you agree that it's your responsibility to check with your GP before taking part in any diet or weight loss program.

This works for **both men and women** but you will have to adjust it accordingly to you and how your body takes to the changes.

This nutrition plan is generic in its nature and not a personalised plan. Therefore this guide doesn't take any medical conditions or health issues you may have into consideration. Please consult your GP and adjust accordingly.

Your results may vary.

By starting this plan you understand, accept and agree that Ben Hulme, The Boot Camper and other associated brands takes no responsibility for any negative effects this has on your health. You also acknowledge that Ben Hulme, The Boot Camper and other associated brands takes no responsibility for the actions of any businesses or products recommended in this guide.

By starting this program, you also understand, accept and agree that this is entirely your decision to start and you take responsibility for your own health.

By using this information, you do so at your own risk.

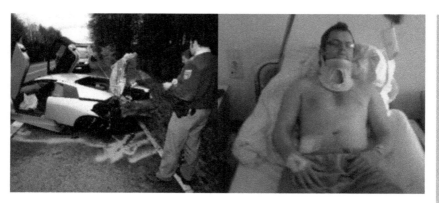

My near death experience. I broke my neck and nearly died as a passenger in a Lamborghini that lost control and hit a tree!

Who am I and why am I qualified to share this with you?

My name is Ben Hulme and after I broke and dislocated my neck in a massive car accident (as a passenger in a Lamborghini) a few years ago, I put on a lot of weight during my 2 year recovery.

I was in Germany at the time of the accident and I had a 6 hour operation to fix my neck. I now have a metal plate, bone from my hip and 4 pins fusing C3 and C4 together.

It was scary and my neurosurgeon said that I was a 'miracle case' and that I should do something with my life as this is my second chance. I will never forget him saying that to me. I am very lucky to be here.

I couldn't do anything physical while I recovered so I ended up becoming really depressed and it pains me to say it, but I turned to junk food for comfort.

As a result, I put on a lot of weight and got myself into a really bad rut. I couldn't blame anyone but myself. I wasn't in a good place at all and I just couldn't seem to shift the weight.

I had a beer belly, 'man boobs' and very low self-esteem. I am very open about what happened and I actually ended up on antidepressants and stomach acid pills to control my acid reflux.

I hated the way I looked. I hated who I had become. I had let myself go – **BIG TIME!**

Everyone could see it. I knew it. But I couldn't admit it.

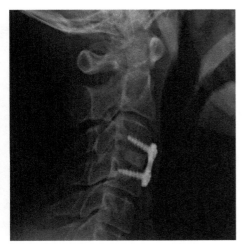

I had C3 and C4 fused together with a metal plate and pins

I lost everything, my daughters, my home, my dream life in Spain and my business. Literally everything I had been working for and built up was gone. I was broken.

It was probably the worst time of my life and I'm not ashamed to admit that I had a full on breakdown.

It was brutal. I have never felt so low, but I knew that things could only get better from that point and I never gave up hope that I would still be able to give my daughters the best life possible.

After a couple of months, things changed and my two daughters came to live with me full-time. I was the happiest man alive!

They have been living with me ever since and that was it, I had to sort myself out to become the best version of myself for them so I really got serious about my health and fitness.

Single parenting can be tough but I knew that if I was to be the best Dad to my daughters I had to focus on my health and that's when my world changed. No more messing about, no more fad diets. I had to sort my life out.

So I started to really learn about food and how it can be used as a tool to get what we want from our bodies and that was the light-bulb moment.

Since that moment, I dabbled with many diets but couldn't ever find something that was sustainable, something that would keep the weight off but allow me to enjoy food!

This went on for years. I just couldn't find anything that I wanted to do long term. It was frustrating. Maybe that's where you are now? I know a lot of my boot campers have told me that they're frustrated with their relationship with food and fad diets.

Then everything changed for me.

The real catalyst that triggered my total body transformation was when my fiancée left me. I won't go into details about that as it's personal, but I hit rock bottom.

I discovered that eating doesn't have to be for pleasure only.

You can eat to get results and eat to literally transform your body once you actually understand how it works.

So I ditched the fad diets and I started my own nutrition plan which I have stuck to sustainably for many years now.

I no longer take any antidepressants and it's been years since I touched any sort of antacid tablets or good old Gaviscon. I have zero acid reflux issues and more energy than I know what to do with!

Exercise and healthy eating has literally become my medicine. The key to health and happiness is within us all, we just have to learn how to achieve it for ourselves and that's what I am going to share with you now.

I'm so blessed to be in a position to help you with your body transformation. As a full-time single father I had to find a way to make an income around my commitments to my daughters, so I studied to become a personal trainer to help others with their body transformations and then I started my boot camps.

I started this from literally zero and I have now trained thousands of boot campers. I am super proud of that and I am beyond proud of them.

If you're anything like me, you are probably very busy. Work, kids and general life can often create hurdles when it comes to your own body transformation.

I have heard it all before and being busy is not an excuse, you can still make this work. I am proof of that!

This whole program has been designed for busy people like us! It's real because I do it, have done it and many others are currently getting insane results from this too.

If you're anything like me, you probably don't have the time or the desire to be spending your valuable time weighing food, scanning barcodes into an app or counting calories etc. So let's scrap that idea right now, you don't need to.

You probably don't want to do anything that involves attending weight-loss groups where you have to weigh-in every week in front of complete strangers! So you can scrap that idea too.

That's not for me! I just don't get it personally...

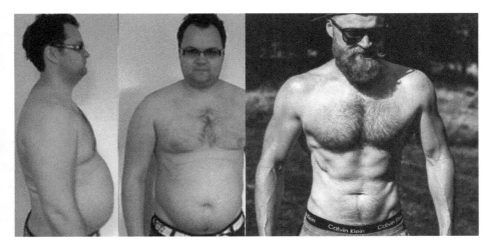

It irritates me that people go to a 'weigh-in' to celebrate losing 1lb or get super down about gaining 1lb. You can't move forward like that, sure there are exceptions, but in reality weight has so many factors that affect it such as hormones, water retention, menstrual cycle, bowel movements etc.

Why waste time worrying about what you have lost or gained every day? It's literally irrelevant and it is actually really damaging to your progress.

I won't go into a massive rant about it, but a little later in this guide I will explain real measurements that will keep you committed and keep you on track. My advice right now is to throw away the scales, smash them up and take a huge sense of pride in doing so! They won't help you, trust me.

Anyway, as I was saying, I am just a normal guy and I believe this is why many people love what I have created because most of us just want to get the results without doing anything too extreme.

We're normal people, not competitive athletes. We just want to feel healthier, look better and fit into our clothes again! Don't worry, you will get there for sure, just stick with me. I am a man with a plan!

I highly recommend that you use this nutrition plan alongside a decent exercise regime so that you achieve the best results possible. For example you could combine this with my workout videos from **TheBootCamper.com**

This is my online video platform, which I designed to help you achieve huge results with your body transformation as if I am training you personally.

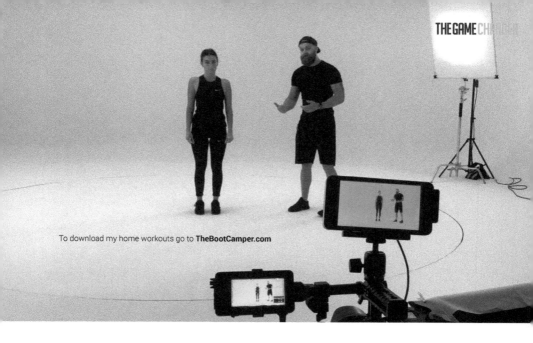

To download my home workouts go to **TheBootCamper.com**

Essentially it's me training you just like we do in my boot camps – but with the added benefit of doing it in the comfort of your own home, anywhere in the world at any time you want.

Plus, to help you further you can access my growing 'inner circle' support community to help you every step of the way so that you get the results you want.

You can access my support community at: **BenHulme.com/mentoring**

Alongside exercising and eating according to this guide, making small changes to your everyday life, like walking more instead of driving everywhere will massively help you achieve results faster.

It all adds up and it's important to commit to this new lifestyle to not only look better, but feel better both physically and mentally. Trust me it's worth it. You will feel absolutely amazing I guarantee it.

I recommend you get a smart watch such as a Fitbit or a Garmin (I personally have a Garmin) and make sure you hit your steps every day, it'll make a massive difference.

There are so many to choose from but it was a game changer for me as I could immediately track my activity.

Recommended:

Fitbit: BenHulme.com/fitbit
Garmin: BenHulme.com/garmin

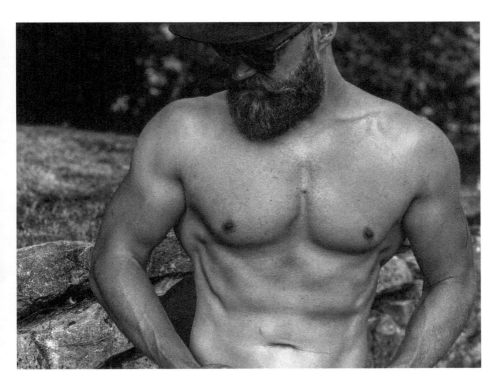

You should aim to exercise 3 to 4 times a week minimum. I do that personally and wouldn't want it any other way.

I feel amazing and so can you. But remember, I didn't start like this it just became my lifestyle over time and I can't recommend it highly enough.

I started out by walking every day for 40 minutes. That in turn got me into other types of training and over time I got the fitness bug.

I'd love for you to share your success story with me. You can either email me or send me a direct message on my social media accounts.

I know that this will literally be life changing if you want it to be and you never know, you could soon be inspiring others too. It's the best feeling ever.

Just remember, I have your back and I am here to help you so let me know if you have any questions and I will do everything I can to help you.

THE
BOOT
CAMPER

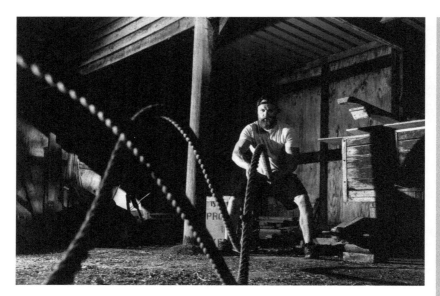

The key to success: Mindset

I strongly believe that the key to success with a body transformation and living a healthy lifestyle is your MINDSET.

To me this is more important than exercise, nutrition or anything else.

It's something most 'diet programs' and so called 'experts' don't help you with, they just get straight into the exercise and nutrition. But because I have done this myself I know what it takes and that's why this guide will have a heavy focus on mindset to start with. It's that important!

One of the main things that could potentially slow up your results is your mindset and it's a huge reason why so many people fail and then put the 'weight' back on again!

It's quite likely that there is a battle going on in your head right now. You want to lose the fat but the instant satisfaction you get when you eat the wrong things always gets in the way. I know it does, I was there.

This is pretty normal, It's because most of us have a sugar addiction and we don't even know it. You're not alone. There is nothing wrong with you. We just have to make you want to achieve your body transformation goals more than anything else.

I've helped so many people now and it's your turn next.

But...

The key to success: Mindset

You have to want to do this.

You have to really want to transform your body, you have to want to get healthy or you won't see the best results.

The key is to ALWAYS focus on the end result and stick to the plan to be sure that you see it through. Commit. Be relentless and I guarantee you will see the results you desire.

Focus on the NOW. The past is done, we can create the future but the NOW is all we have. You can become whoever you want to be and look however you want to look. You can and will become the best version of yourself, why wouldn't you want that?

It does get a lot easier as the weeks go on because you become more efficient, more healthy and more confident in yourself. So stick with it, and ride it out if it's tough at first, which it could well be.

Let it happen though. Don't hold back and don't hesitate. This WILL become a reality for you.

As I say, you must be in the 'NOW' and only look forward. Always ask yourself if what you are doing right NOW will take you towards your goals or away from them?

If you can't answer 'towards my goals' then you're doing something wrong. Don't worry, we're only human but give yourself a metaphorical slap on the wrist and change what you're doing so that you're only working towards your goals not against them, unless it's a cheat meal, then don't worry at all just enjoy yourself (more about cheat meals later!).

Don't ever stop until you reach your goals. Make it happen. Don't ever give up because I promise you, being fit, healthy and confident in your own skin is the best feeling ever.

It will get easier so stick to the plan and as your sugar addiction slows down, you will find that it becomes easier as the cravings subside.

This all starts with your mindset because your brain is the most powerful organ when it comes to your success with this. No, not your stomach! It's your brain and ultimately that boils down to your mindset.

THE BOOT CAMPER

All the cravings, the sugar addiction and the desire to eat the wrong things come from your brain. So if you are able to control your brain and your mindset then you will find this so much easier.

Your healthy lifestyle efforts need to be built on solid foundations not on quicksand or you will be destined to fail.

So how does this mindset thing work?

You have to know in your heart of hearts that you are going to transform your body. Believe me when I say that this works and let me be the first to reassure and guarantee that if you follow what I am going to share with you in this book, you will transform your body. It's actually impossible not to.

Start believing in yourself and your ability to make this finally work for you. This is the answer you have been looking for. The key to your success. I have proven it myself, with my boot campers and now, with you.

If you don't believe it, then it will never happen. You have to know from your very core that this is what you want to do. You have to understand you will have some tough times, you will have moments where you want to quit, but you have to stay focused, stay committed and be relentless in your quest to transform your body!

You're human. You will make mistakes. You will mess up, but remember this is **LONG TERM** not a quick fix. This isn't another yo-yo diet that promises the world and under-delivers.

You can go as extreme as you want with this plan, but I repeat, you will get the best results if you stick to this to the letter – **GUARANTEED!**

The reason this works and the reason you will get results with this is the fact that it's all about how we are designed to eat but remember that you have to be 'in it to win it' or it simply won't work!

You can do what most people do and tell the world you're on a diet by posting photos of your food and your new healthy lifestyle on social media and that's great for accountability, but if you are secretly stuffing your face with chocolate biscuits when you're alone, the only person you are letting down is YOURSELF.

You are in fact lying to yourself and that's not OK. It's weird, but some people actually self-sabotage their efforts but pretend to be committed.

You either want this or you don't.

The sad reality is no one else really gives a cr*p about your diet (there you go I said it!), they only really care about themselves – so you must do this for **YOURSELF** because it's what **YOU** want to do.

The key to success: Mindset

Dedicate yourself to this and you will see epic results. Not just small results, but noticeable results that will get people asking how you did it.

BUT BE AWARE: Many people will try to bring you down, many of your friends and even your family may try to convince you to stop with your health journey and try to convince you to eat how they eat.

This is because everyone thinks that their way of eating is correct because no one likes to be in the wrong. It's almost a taboo subject that people don't want to discuss even when they know they are in the wrong.

By taking action and committing to changing your body, you are potentially and inadvertently highlighting other people's own insecurities with their bodies and that often makes them feel uncomfortable.

So instead of supporting you they will often try to pull you down and get you to quit and therefore fail. It's very normal, it happened to me and I see it all the time.

Sick isn't it?

But that's the way it works sometimes. I still get it now! You just have to keep strong and continue as planned because this is your body and your life, not anyone else's.

The ironic thing is that when you have had success with this, they will soon be asking you how you did it! Just send them my way OK?!

Many of my friends and even some of my family members say things like "why are you eating healthy all the time? We are all going to die one day anyway" and things like, "you could be hit by a bus tomorrow! You might as well enjoy food, life's too short".

Don't listen to them.

Being healthy helps you to live a happier, more fulfilled life so stick to the plan because it's going to be a game changer.

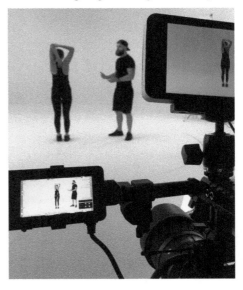

For home based workouts join
TheBootCamper.com

The irony is that I love what I eat and believe me, I eat lots.

By eating healthy we are increasing our chances of living longer, decreasing our chances of disease and ultimately we will be able to enjoy our lives more. We have more energy, we can think clearer and we are way more productive. Plus, statistically it's unlikely we will 'get hit by a bus tomorrow'.

So don't base your future health and happiness on what others say when they try to bring you down because they know they should in fact be doing the same as you. Crazy isn't it.

I even had one friend throwing chocolates at me the other day when I was having a healthy lunch. He was trying to get me to 'break', eat the chocolate and give up on my health journey!

Needless to say, it didn't work. It just highlighted to me that people will always try to hold you back if they aren't actually happy with their own bodies.

The reality is that if I saw someone eating healthy and trying to better themselves why on earth would I want to stop them? See what I'm trying to say? It's madness and only a reflection on their own unhappiness with their body image.

Listen to me when I say that YOU CAN do this. No matter what your current situation is, no matter what your friends or family say, you can make this happen. You can get healthy, lose fat, gain confidence and ultimately be happy. In fact, I guarantee it.

If you are stuck at any point head to **BenHulme.com/mentoring** and get the full support membership to get the help, support and motivation from our other members and myself within our support community.

We are all on the same journey as you and would never dream of holding you back!

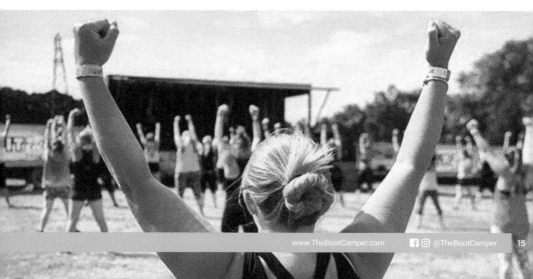

Leverage compound interest

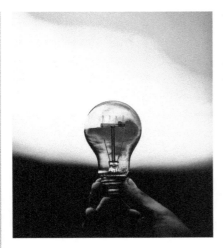

If you aren't familiar with the term 'compound interest' I want to open your mind to this concept with regards to your body transformation.

Put simply: one burger won't make you fat and equally one salad won't make you thin! But it's what we do daily over time that determines the outcome of our efforts.

From now on we will be focusing on leveraging compound interest.

This means that we will be eating the correct foods in the knowledge that over time our efforts will compound to create the results we desire.

Think about what you are doing daily towards the end result you desire. As I said before, remember to live in the 'now' and consider if this takes you towards or away from what you are trying to achieve.

The fact is that it's just as easy to have a healthy meal as it is to have an unhealthy one. It's the same process of putting food in your mouth! It's the small efforts that we make daily that determine what our bodies look like on the outside and how they perform on the inside.

We literally are what we eat so let's fuel our bodies correctly. Let's eat what we are designed to eat and over time we will become the very best versions of ourselves.

We aren't designed to eat most of the food that we consume these days. That's part of the problem, we all have an addiction to sugar and processed food.

So when you change your diet and eat the way I am about to show you in this guide, you will reset your body and it will perform how it's designed to perform. This is simply because you will be fueling it with what it's designed to be fueled by. Makes sense right?!

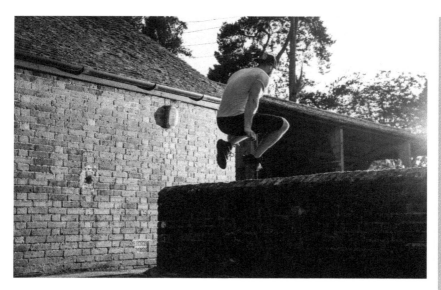

Our bodies

No matter what we look like, we have been given a gift.

We are alive and we have beautiful bodies that deserve to be looked after and not neglected.

The thought of death scares most people, so why are we pumping our bodies full of cr*p that won't help us to be as healthy as we can be? Why are we eating things that we know can cause diseases and obesity? We are self-sabotaging. Why?

We all know that health is the most important thing. Well, it would seem that most people don't think so at all. Just look around you, just look at what people eat these days, is it even food?!

Sure, unhealthy food and drink can taste amazing and it makes us feel good in the short term, but what is it doing to our bodies long term? Remember, compound interest! You have a choice right now.

Don't lie to yourself and eat the bad food assuming it's not going to be a problem because it adds up and over time it can make you really ill. Keep it healthy and learn to love this new lifestyle because your body will love you for it.

Remember, one burger won't make you fat! But eating badly every meal will! You'll discover 'cheat meals' within this nutrition plan. They will help you to commit and stay on track long term to see the results that you desire.

Our bodies

Imagine your body is a race engine. Stop feeding it with low-grade fuel. Start feeding it with the very best fuel possible if you want to perform the best you possibly can. Feed yourself with race fuel!

We all want the best out of life don't we? We all want to look good, feel good, be happier, perform better, have more energy, have better relationships, be more productive, live longer etc. But far too many people expect that high performance but they continue to use low-grade fuel!

What baffles me is that people struggle to drink enough water every day yet they happily drink 8 pints of lager on a Friday night without thinking twice! Seriously?!

The funny thing is, I can say this because that was the old me! I was feeding myself badly with the wrong fuel for many years and that compounded into me becoming overweight and depressed. I changed it and you can too.

This is your body, not anyone else's. No one is going to make this happen for you. To change your life you need to make life-changing decisions and that starts now!

By leveraging compound interest the results will be clear. So much so that you will never want to go back to how you were before. Believe me, it's so much better living life like this. Chase it down for yourself as you will love the new improved version of yourself.

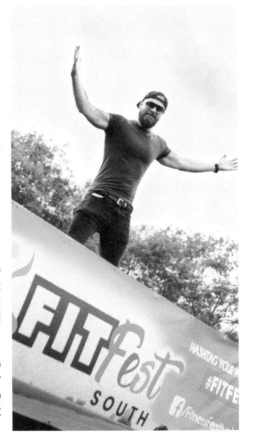

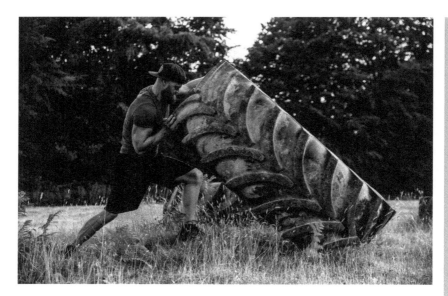

This isn't 'rocket science', it's just a case of doing what's right for our bodies before it's too late. Don't look back with regret when you get sick wishing you had done more sooner. We aren't designed to live forever so remember my slogan... Life's short, live well!

You're clearly motivated to transform your body which is why you have purchased this book. BUT, what happens when that motivation goes?

What happens when you are having an off day?

Believe me, I've had many days during my journey where I have felt super unmotivated. We're only human right?

But luckily for you I have worked out the best ways to keep going and stay motivated without quitting and giving up.

The main thing I found motivating was visualizing where I wanted to be. Focusing on what I would look like and feel like when I achieved my goals.

What I discovered is that with each week that passed I felt better and better. It became almost addictive and over time I found that I didn't want to go back to my old habits and unhealthy ways.

Motivation

Here are some accountability steps you should take, starting now:

Take a 'BEFORE' photo!

I started this whole journey by taking a 'before' photo. I took a few and promised myself that I would never look like that again.

I recommend that you do the same. Take a photo of yourself today. You can keep this as a reminder of what the 'old you' looked like and it's a great reference point to see how far you've come.

You don't need to post it online and you don't need to send it to me, just keep it for your records. It will massively help motivate you and show you how far you have come with your body transformation.

Set up a private Instagram account

You can take photos of your meals and selfie style photos and videos to keep a record of what you are doing and how you feel etc. Just like a diary or a journal. I personally found it very useful in the early stages and it kept me motivated to keep going.

It's handy to use Instagram as a hub so that your photos and videos are all in one place in chronological order without being mixed up with the other photos on your phone, camera or computer.

It's effectively your log of your body transformation journey.

You can also 'pay it forward' and use your journey to inspire other people and I welcome you to follow and tag my account: **Instagram.com/thebootcamper** or use the **#TheBootCamper** hashtag within your instagram photos on your account.

You can also follow and tag my personal account too: **Intagram.com/benhulme** and tag **#BenHulmeFitness**

Clothing

One of the best ways to gauge your progress and to motivate yourself is to measure how your clothing fits. Find an old item of clothing that you used to fit into, or go to the shop and buy something new that you would like to fit into (something that would make you feel amazing!) and keep going until you reach that goal.

Your existing clothing is also a great way to gauge your progress as it will become baggier and fit you differently (or not fit you at all soon).

The clothing doesn't lie, whereas the scales may give you a false reading of your success. So use clothes as a fantastic guide, you will know when you are seeing success, trust me. I had to buy a whole new wardrobe when I went from a 38" waist to a 32".

It's a great feeling! Make it happen.

Am I happy naked?

YES REALLY! One of the best things I also found for motivation was to wake up in the morning and stand in front of the mirror completely naked, yep!

I would then ask myself a simple question "Am I happy with my body?"

If I answered 'no' then I knew I had to keep going. This is a powerful way to do it and when you start answering 'yes' and seeing the results you desire it's a wonderful feeling. You will notice small changes over time. Muscles showing up where you haven't seen them before, just stare at yourself and be grateful for this journey you are on. Take a moment to think about the day ahead and promise yourself that you will get through the day and commit to the plan.

Whatever you do don't 'hate' the way you are now. I hear that a lot.

It's not good. You got yourself to this point. Leverage it. Accept and embrace it and move forward. You should be very proud of yourself for taking the action required to change your body and ultimately your life.

Regrets from your deathbed

As you know, because I nearly died in a car accident I find that I have a slightly different outlook on life to many other people. I often think about my future because I have had a second chance to live my life.

I think about my future self looking back from my deathbed and I ask myself "did I do everything I could do to live the best life I could live? Did I do everything I could to be healthy in order to live as long as possible? Did I do everything I could to be the best Dad and role model to my daughters?"

The reason that this works for me, is that I don't want to leave this life as a disappointment to myself (or anyone else for that matter). I want to be sure that I did everything I could do to be the best I could possibly be. Not just for myself but for my friends, my family, my boot campers and you!

Motivation

Just think about when you're old and you look back on your life. That will be you one day. Do you want to lie there with regret that you didn't do everything you could to live the best life possible? Do you want to be angry with yourself because you didn't take charge of your health when you had the chance?

You don't know why you will be on your deathbed. No one does until they are there, so why not give yourself the best chance to be the best you, the healthiest version of you so that you can really live your very best life.

Many people would argue that making money is the most important thing, but making money should never be at the detriment of your health. No one wants to be the richest man in the graveyard. Money can't save you and you can't take it with you. Time ticks away and we can't stop it. So health is all we really have, therefore health is wealth!!

No matter what shape or size you are I guarantee that there is someone out there who would literally love to have a body like yours.

Never take what you have for granted, this is just the beginning and learn to be happy with where you are now, safe in the knowledge that you're improving and becoming healthier.

We all have one shot at this so please make it count. You owe it to yourself.

Stop weighing yourself

Please stop weighing yourself every day. It's misleading and it's dangerous for your mindset.

The scales are the enemy!

Weigh yourself after 6 months if you have to. But my best advice is to go on other measurements such as a before photo or how your clothing fits etc. This is far more accurate unless you're a boxer trying to 'make weight' or you are about to jump out of a plane for example!

Of course you will want to know how you're progressing but the scales are possibly the worst and most irrelevant way to do this. The next time someone asks what you 'weigh' take pride in saying that you don't know or care what you weigh because it's irrelevant.

THE
BOOT
CAMPER

I genuinely have no clue what I weigh right now. In fact I don't care! I know I'm actually getting heavier because while I'm losing fat, I'm gaining muscle. Muscle is denser than fat so in turn my weight is actually going up even though I am getting leaner.

So if I was to measure my success on weight alone it would make me feel like I am doing something wrong and that's because we are conditioned to think that we need to 'weigh less' to be healthier, which isn't necessarily true.

Body fat percentage is the real measurement but we don't all have the ability to measure that, so we need to go on what we can measure such as clothing or photos for example as I mentioned before.

Too many people weigh themselves literally every single day and they get upset or unmotivated if they haven't lost any weight that day. It's ridiculous because there are so many factors that affect weight loss or weight gain in a twenty-four hour period especially for women.

When I started doing longer-term weight loss and living a healthy lifestyle I didn't weigh myself for 6 months. It was amazing to see the results over a longer period of time. Combined with the 'before' photo, the clothing and other measurements it's incredible to see the transformation. I recommend you do the same.

Move past the past

Don't let previous 'failed diets' or your lack of 'time' or 'motivation' stop you or hold you back. The only person who can make this happen is YOU. So make your future self proud. You'll thank yourself one day I guarantee it.

Please don't let bad or negative previous experiences slow you down because you now have the secret to totally transform your body. I guarantee that you will feel absolutely amazing once you start to see the results from this unique nutrition plan.

Don't forget to become a full member of our inner circle support community at **BenHulme.com/mentoring** to keep yourself motivated.

We are doing this as a team and we share food photos, recipes and motivate each other as a community.

You are welcome to join us, in fact I recommend it. As a family we will help you every step of the way and hopefully you will help to inspire others too with your success from this.

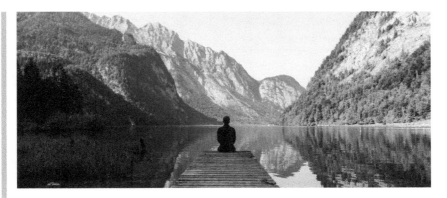

Focusing on positives is really important. You should never focus on the negatives. Stop feeling sorry for yourself, stop telling yourself how big you are or how fat you feel etc. This isn't healthy. You will learn that you need to be happy with yourself now.

Accept yourself for who you are. You got yourself here, take responsibility for it, own it, it's no one else's fault. Don't blame others. You can't blame your friends, your family, your parents, the kids etc.

This is YOU and it's down to you! But the exciting part is that this is the worst it's going to get. You can only improve from here. If you use this to your advantage this will change your life just like it has mine!

Remember to take your 'before' photo and promise yourself that you will never go back to how you are now. Set that promise in concrete and let's smash it.

Everything that you have done in your life so far has got you to this point and things are going to get better from now onwards.

By looking down on yourself negatively though, you will be thinking in a backwards motion.

You will be focusing on what's been done and how you got there. You can't move forwards looking backwards so you now need to focus on the future and think in a forward motion so that you can work towards where you want to be.

You are incredible. Don't let anyone ever tell you different. You owe it to yourself to think positively and move forward towards your goals with a huge confident smile. You are going to become the best version of you and that's something to celebrate.

Thinking positively is really important for your journey. Think about how good you will feel when people comment on your new improved body because it will happen I guarantee it.

Believe me it feels awesome when you get to that point and it will happen for you, but only if you want it to!

These are fundamental parts to your success with this. It's a very important lesson because negatives will only bring about more of that negativity. So you need to be positive and focus only on achieving that end result.

We are all energy and negativity attracts more negativity. Positivity attracts more positivity. What you choose to attract is 100% down to you and your mindset. Don't believe me? Just look at my story.

When I was overweight and in a negative space, everything went wrong for me. Now look what's happened since I decided to focus on myself and think positively. My whole world changed and yours can too.

Just sit back for a second and imagine what it feels like to be the size you want to be. Imagine what it feels like to be on the beach feeling super confident about your body. Feels good right? Now let's make that a reality for you.

Put it like this...

It can't get any worse than it is right now can it? You have committed to a plan that genuinely works and is now getting results for people daily! This will work for you too.

You now have your hands on the last nutrition plan you will ever need because this is 100% sustainable and I know that first hand as I have done this day in day out for many years. It's not called the Game Changer for nothing and now it's your turn!

Don't forget that you can compliment this nutrition plan with my home based workout videos at **TheBootCamper.com** so that you can set up your own boot camps at home.

It's a proven exercise regime to go with this nutrition plan and you can also access our growing inner circle support community via **BenHulme. com/mentoring** to help you every step of the way.

So go get it! Become the best version of yourself and celebrate what's about to happen to your mindset and your body.

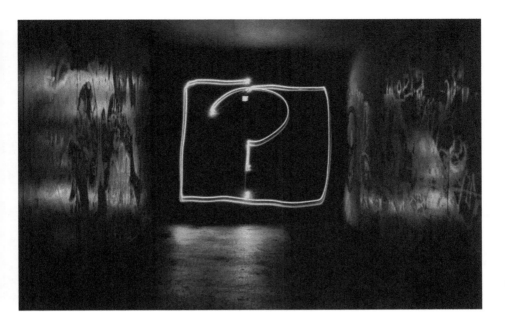

So how does this work?

The secret to this working is for you to be in a daily calorie deficit. That means you need to burn more calories than you consume in a day. That's the secret and in this chapter you will discover why.

Most people are living their lives permanently in a calorie surplus where they are consuming more calories than they burn. This simply means that you will put on fat!

So by living in a calorie deficit we are forcing our bodies to burn the fat. Now it's a little more complicated than this but it's important to know that you will be using food as a tool to literally force your body to transform into the best version of yourself.

The body is designed to adapt to its environment. We are very clever animals. We can adapt to whatever environment we are put in. It's important to force that change on our bodies in order to get the results we desire.

Eating 'healthy' sounds a bit boring right? But what if I was to say that eating how we are designed to eat will...

• **Change your life**
• **Transform your body**
• **Increase your energy levels**
• **Boost your immune system**
• **Enable you to think clearer**
• **Live with a more positive mindset**

Sounds good right?

Listen, I literally don't care about any of these big diet companies (I won't name names) that promise fast results and force you to count calories using a points system because they are simply very clever businesses.

They work to a point because the system they use gets you to cut calories. Of course you are going to 'lose weight' because your body will adapt, but then you will most definitely plateau quite quickly. This is when the problem starts and the weight goes back on. I hear it time and time again.

This is because these companies have 'educated' (brainwashed) you into believing that certain foods are OK because you use a points system. This means that you can pretty much eat what you want as long as it's within your allocated points. So therefore a lot of the food you crave is OK as long as you eat a controlled portion of it.

So the issue here is that this means you will assume that it's going to be a good thing to eat this long term. It's not.

Once you see the results from these types of 'diets', you will continue to eat the foods you crave because you have been 'advised' that they are good for you. Then, because you are happy with the results the portion sizes slowly and steadily become bigger again and you stop with the calorie counting and what happens next?

You put the weight back on only to re-join their 'diet club' and start the whole process again.

These diets are not healthy. Sustainable body transformations take time and if done correctly there is absolutely no reason for the fat to go back on.

What people are forgetting is the visceral fats. That's the internal fats that surround some of your major internal organs. So when those friends of yours say that it doesn't matter what they eat because they just don't get fat, they are possibly not as healthy as they make out. That's because they could have a super high visceral fat percentage and that's potentially lethal.

This nutrition plan will also help to break down the visceral fats as well as external fats because you will be eating 'healthy' not by a points system that lets you eat what you want while cutting calories. Don't believe the hype.

So how does this works?

These companies are not educating you about what your body is actually designed to eat. They are simply running a clever business that feeds off of the extreme success stories from some members to motivate you to get results. But because you aren't being educated about what's actually good and what's not you will nearly always put the fat back on and end up 'yo-yo' dieting!

Why is an avocado more 'points' than some chocolate bars according to these diet companies? Come on, avocados are awesome!

You'll find that you keep going around in circles. You lose the weight, you plateau and then you put the weight back on only to then come back to their clever business to do it all again.

Listen to me. Don't lie to yourself, you know this is true but that's all about to change as you are about to get an education in eating how we are designed to eat and discover exactly how to lose the weight, keep it off and transform your body to become the ultimate version of yourself.

A lot of people don't realise that you can actually eat differently to achieve different results. You can eat to be healthy, eat to grow bigger and more muscular, eat to lose body fat, eat to put on fat, in fact we can do whatever we want with food because as I said before, our clever bodies are designed to adapt.

So when you eat a certain way, the laws of compound interest come into play and we adapt over time. So the question is: How do we force our body to drop the unwanted body fat, tone up and totally transform?

The answer is simple:

1. **You speed up your metabolism**
2. **Drink more water**
3. **Minimise blood-sugar spikes**
4. **Eat in a calorie deficit**
5. **Increase your protein intake**
6. **Eat carbs at the right times**

That right there is the secret to success!

This means that you won't go hungry because you will be eating more often.

In fact you should be eating a really decent amount of food every few hours in the day. This means that your stomach will nearly always have food in it.

By consuming the right foods at the right times we will become the best versions of ourselves. But by over consuming the wrong foods and living in a calorie surplus (consuming more calories than we burn) we force our bodies to store energy in the form of glycogen which ultimately makes us bigger.

THE BOOT CAMPER

Our bodies store this glycogen in our livers, our muscles and some in adipose tissue, all of which have limited storage. But if we consume too many carbs and they aren't burnt off they're converted into fat, of which we have unlimited storage. So, the longer we stay in a calorie surplus the longer we are going to continue to put on fat.

But it's a little more complicated than that because it comes down to carbohydrates and our blood-sugar levels.

You see there is a common myth about carbs. People assume that to transform your body we need to drop all carbs! It's myth. I mean, of course you would lose 'weight' because for every 1 gram of glycogen stored we also store 2-4 grams of water. So there would of course be a quick weight drop due to 'water weight' but you will also have very little energy so how can you truly transform your body without the energy necessary to do so?

To truly transform your body you need to workout. You can't properly transform your body without some form of exercise, you can only go so far with diet alone. But to workout you definitely need energy so you can't just drop the carbs completely!

The thing is that there are many diet plans out there. Of course some of them work to a point, but you want to transform your body forever and never go back to where you are now right? You want to become the best version of yourself, the fittest and the healthiest you can be?

Then you will definitely need to eat carbs! But you need to consume the right carbs at the right times. That's the difference. More about carbs later in this book.

It's super important to realise that:

1. CARBS ARE ENERGY
2. PROTEIN IS REPAIR

We need the carbs as energy to function properly and then we need the protein to repair and sustain our bodies development. Both carbs and protein are the key to success with your body transformation, which I will explain in more detail a little later.

I imagine that if you are anything like me you are pretty excited to hear that you can transform your body and eat carbs. I love carbs!!

Alongside speeding up our metabolism we need to manage our blood-sugar levels and avoid blood-sugar spikes by consuming the right carbohydrates at the right times and by consuming less sugary food and drink.

So how does this works?

The science behind this:

There is a science behind this and here is the simple version for you.

Most people constantly feed their bodies with fast-acting carbs and sugary foods. When we do this we effectively have instant energy (you can see it in kids when they eat sugary food because they instantly go hyper. I know my daughters do).

This is because these fast-acting carbs spike our blood-sugar levels and the problem is that when we have all that energy and we don't burn it off we ultimately store it as 'glycogen' in our fat reserves.

The storage of glycogen starts in our liver and our muscles, adipose and then our fat reserves. The liver and our muscles have limited storage but our fat reserves have unlimited storage so when we consume too many calories and don't burn them off they are stored and that is what makes us 'fat'.

So how do we force our bodies to change this?

The real magic happens when we manage our blood-sugar levels by eliminating the fast-acting carbs and sugary foods.

This forces our bodies to get the energy from our fat reserves and forces our pancreas to release a peptide hormone called 'glucagon'.

Glucagon stimulates the release of glycogen (stored energy) therefore increasing our blood glucose levels so that we have the energy we need. It works in the opposite way to the hormone 'insulin' which lowers our blood sugar levels when it's too high (you will have heard of insulin when talking about diabetes).

By avoiding blood-sugar spikes we are forcing our bodies to release the stored glycogen as a source of energy. It's what we are designed to do and over time this results in a rapid loss of fat in our bodies.

It's a simple science but it's important to understand that our bodies are in a permanent state of 'homeostasis' which means that we are automatically, constantly trying to find the perfect balance.

We have a very clever hormonal system called the 'Endocrine System' that's always working to make sure that our bodies are functioning to their best.

Makes sense right? If not don't panic. It works. Just go with it...!

THE
BOOT
CAMPER

THE GAME CHANGER

Eat more not less...

It's a complete myth that you need to eat less to transform your body. It's funny because a lot of people ask me what I eat to be in decent shape and they assume that I eat next to nothing and live on kale shakes! I eat like a horse. I am always eating. I love food. You need to eat more not less, but more of the right stuff!

Eating less will slow down your metabolism and over time will force you to put on weight. It's really weird I know but to be healthy you need to eat little and often.

The way I have structured this nutrition plan means that you can live a very normal life with your regular three meals a day. This means that you can be social and have breakfast, lunch and dinner just like everyone else but the difference is that you will need to have 2-3 additional snacks in between these meals.

It's fantastic because you get to eat a lot and transform your body!

The plan of action

This isn't like other 'diet plans', this is the Game Changer and the good thing is that this means we get to eat a decent amount of food.

This may sound crazy because there is a common misconception that to lose fat you shouldn't eat very much. But in reality it's super important that you eat often to speed up your metabolism and not hold onto fat as 'stored energy'.

This is what will get the results and transform your body.

With the Game Changer you will have three meals like normal, this is what makes it sustainable because you can live a 'normal' life and eat at normal times like everyone else.

The difference is that you will have snacks in between these meals to ensure that you are eating often. This means that you are going to be constantly fueling your body with food to speed up your metabolism.

You will now be eating the right food, quality food, the food we are actually designed to eat! Race fuel.

This is how you will be eating from now on and I guarantee it will transform your body.

In the next few pages you will discover a list of what you need to eat for each meal and for each snack. This is essential, but it gives you the flexibility to adapt it to your own tastes and dietary requirements.

You can be as strict as you want with this. However, if you go 100% on plan you will see better and faster results, but the goal is to make this totally sustainable for you.

THE BOOT CAMPER

Meal 1: Breakfast

Protein + unrefined/complex carbs + fats
(Plus multivitamin and Omega 3 pill)

Examples:

- 2 boiled eggs and porridge made with almond milk and a teaspoon of organic honey if necessary

- Porridge with some peanut butter, a banana and a teaspoon of organic honey

- Eggs and half an avocado on one slice of wholemeal bread (no butter)

- Protein shake with pre-ground porridge oats, a banana and some peanut butter (this is my go to and I use a NUTRIBULLET to prepare it).

- Could prepare 'overnight protein oats' the night before. Place oats in a jar with almond milk (or similar), add protein powder and stir. Leave overnight ready to eat in the morning. Can add fruit - it's great!

There are so many options but be sure to have some unrefined/complex carbs and a source of protein + fats for your breakfast.

You need energy for the day so make sure that you don't skip breakfast, it's detrimental to your success with this. If you are busy you can prepare the night before.

Going for such a long time without food will eventually slow your metabolism and you will feel lethargic. We need energy and we get that from carbs and fats and the morning is the perfect time to have this combination.

Take your multivitamin with your breakfast and your Omega 3 pill too.

Snack 1: Mid morning snack

Protein + fats and/or fruit

Examples:

- Half a handful of plain (unsalted/unsweetened) nuts and a piece of fruit

- Some carrot sticks with some hummus

- Protein shake and ground oats with water or almond milk

- Half an avocado and a boiled egg

This first snack is to make sure that you are digesting food between breakfast and lunch. Have something quick and easy so that you don't skip it.

There are loads of options even if you are on the road or sat at your desk at work. Just plan this snack before as it's a very important part of this nutrition plan.

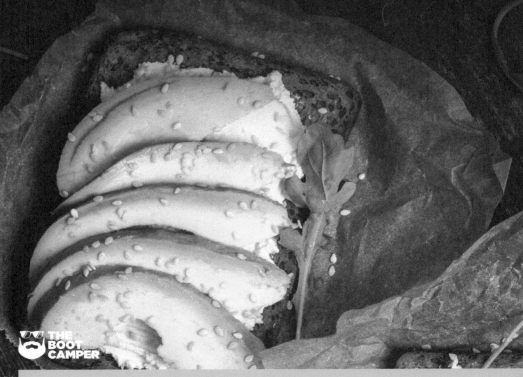

THE
BOOT
CAMPER

Meal 2: Lunch

Protein + unrefined/complex carbs + veggies
Any meat or protein source, any unrefined/complex carb and unlimited veggies/salad.

Examples:

- Chicken breast with sweet potato and steamed veggies

- Chicken thighs with brown rice and oven roasted veggies

- Tuna with quinoa and salad with olive oil, lemon juice and vinegar

- Steamed salmon with whole-grain pasta and salad

- Tofu with steamed veggies and roasted sweet potato

To be honest, there are unlimited options for this just be sure to get the protein, that carb and veggies on your plate. You can flavour the food with herbs and spices to make it taste really lovely.

You can meal prep the night before or even a few days before if you feel that this is going to become an issue to prepare this type of food in the day.

Many people prepare their lunches on a Sunday night ready for the week ahead. Personally I don't meal prep longer than one day ahead, but this is your call.

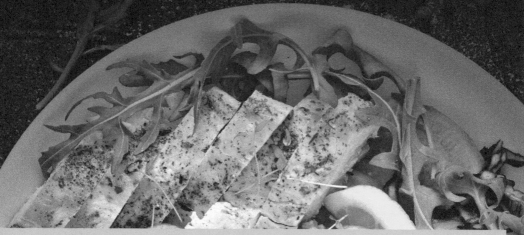

Snack 2: Mid afternoon snack

Protein and unrefined/complex carbs

Examples:

- Same as lunch

- Protein shake with water and some pre-ground oats

- Boiled eggs with raw veggies

- Banana with some peanut butter on rice cakes

- Half a handful of nuts and some fruit

- Biltong (not beef jerky as it's loaded with sugar) and some dried fruit

Unless you are working out later in the evening this will be the last carbs you have for the day.

This snack keeps your body digesting food between lunch and dinner.

This can be the same as meal 2 (lunch) so you could prepare your lunch and then split it into two meals and eat half for lunch and then the second half for your second snack.

Some people find it hard to fit this snack into their day but it's a super important part of this so be sure to prepare it before if necessary.

Meal 3: Dinner

Protein + veggies (no carb for this meal unless immediately after a workout)

Examples:

- Chicken breast with steamed veggies

- Chicken thighs with oven roasted veggies

- Tuna and egg salad with olive oil, lemon juice and vinegar

- Steamed salmon with grilled veggies or salad

- Tofu with steamed veggies

- Steak and oven roasted veggies

- Beef or chicken with stir fried vegetables

The possibilities are endless with this. Remember to use lots of herbs and spices to flavour the food. It doesn't have to be boring.

It's super important to remember NOT to have the carb for this meal because it's the end of the day and you are unlikely to burn that energy off.

The exception to this is if this meal is immediately after a workout. In that case you can time your carbs around your workout. Remember, carbs are energy, but we also need them to restore the glycogen in our muscles which would have depleted during our workout.

We don't need the energy before we go to bed as we won't burn it off. So try to avoid the carb on your last meal of the day. This is a key element to success with fat loss and will massively help you to get the results you desire.

Have this snack ONLY if you are hungry or after working out. Have a whey isolate protein shake with water.

I recommend getting your whey isolate here: **BenHulme.com/protein**

Tip: If you get different flavours, then you have more choice and it will make your snacks more enjoyable. You can also whip up some protein powder with warm water to make an 'angel delight' type desert.

Take it day by day

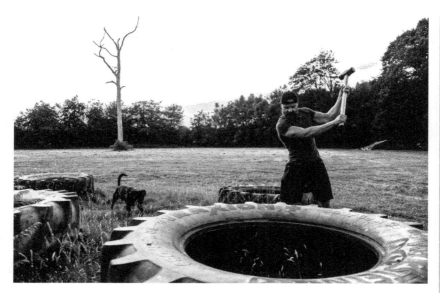

I have structured this nutrition plan so that it's simple to follow and totally sustainable. It enables you to live a completely normal life by eating at the same time others do (breakfast, lunch and dinner).

You won't be doing anything weird, skipping meals, fasting, making lots of juices or shakes and you won't be buying anything from one brand or company making them a lot of money.

This plan has been designed so that you can stay on track from day one.

I have done this for more than 3 years now and I guarantee it works, not only personally but for every single person who commits to making it work. This is totally backed by science and it simply works because it's how we are designed to eat.

Just take it day by day and enjoy the process. It becomes really addictive because you will feel amazing!

Essentials to get started

Here are some essentials that will help you to achieve the ultimate success with this plan.

1. Get a decent multivitamin

This is an essential supplement. You want to make sure that you are getting all the correct vitamins and minerals into your body each day.

Take it each day with your first meal. Multivitamins can make you feel sick if taken on an empty stomach.

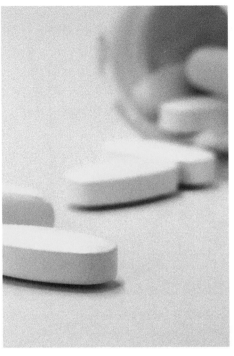

Without a good multivitamin you could potentially be starving your body of essential vitamins it needs to live a healthy life. To get all these vitamins in your body from food and drink alone is very hard. You would need to have a near perfect, super varied diet and that's not always easy to do especially if you are busy.

Taking a multivitamin supplement each day is going to really set you up to achieve your goals and guarantee you are getting your micronutrients.

You can get a good multivitamin from most local health stores or online. Due to the fact that you will consume very little dairy on this nutrition plan I recommend you get yourself a decent multi vitamin with iron and calcium in it (especially for women). Of course you can also get calcium from almond milk, soya milk, or oat milk as they're fortified.

Recommended:
BenHulme.com/vitamin

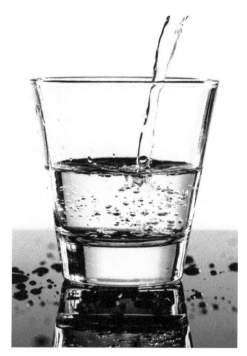

2. Drink a lot more water

Another really important part of this nutrition plan is your consumption of water. You need to make sure that you drink enough!

Try to drink at least two, ideally three litres each and every day.

Water is very important for transforming your body and indeed your health in general because your body uses it in all its cells, organs and tissues to help regulate its temperature and maintain other bodily functions.

Our bodies are made up of 60% water but we lose water through breathing, sweating and digestion so it's super important to drink fluids and to consume foods that contain water to stay hydrated especially if we are exercising regularly **(which you should be doing)**.

You will lose 'water weight' and fat with this plan very quickly. Ironically, drinking more water helps us to lose water weight as our bodies flush it out faster. Water weight is essentially what makes us look bloated so once this has gone we immediately look healthier and 'thinner'. Your skin will also naturally become clearer because you are properly hydrated.

I try to carry a 1.5 litre bottle of water with me most of the time and I aim to finish it twice a day. It's a really easy way to gauge what you are drinking without having to fill a glass up all the time.

Water also helps to flush all the toxins out of your body so it's pretty important to drink plenty of it.

A great tip is to drink a large glass of water first thing in the morning. We have already established that water hydrates you but it has also been scientifically proven to fire up your metabolism, flush toxins from your body and fuel your brain.

The Game Changer: Eat more not less

A lot of people confuse thirst for hunger so they usually eat an unhealthy snack when they are in fact, just thirsty. I was totally guilty of this before I started on my health journey however, as soon as I started drinking more water I noticed an immediate change in the way I was feeling both physically and mentally.

Listen to **YOUR** body though and be sure not to consume too much water as it can actually be harmful to your body. My best advice would be to consume more than you currently do during this plan but don't go over doing it!

Quick Tip:

The fastest and easiest way to tell if you are drinking enough water is to look at your pee. If it is a yellow colour then you are not drinking enough.

You want your urine to be as close to the colour of water as possible. So take a quick glance down at the toilet when you are finished and you can see if you are hydrated or not...

If it's yellow drink more. Simple.

3. Omega 3

Omega 3 is one of the best-researched supplements on earth. It's a daily essential in my honest opinion and something I simply wouldn't be without.

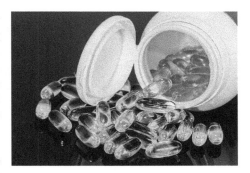

The benefits are huge from helping with our skin, hearts, brain function and even helping with depression, dementia, arthritis, inflammation and so much more.

They also help to lower your blood pressure and they help with your central nervous system which in turn helps you to function better. The list is endless.

I highly recommend you get yourself a good Omega 3 tablet. This will help with your intake of 'good fats' because not all fats are bad.

You will get Omega 3 from fish, some nuts and other 'good' fatty foods but taking an Omega 3 pill as a supplement will directly benefit you and guarantee you are getting what you need into your body each day.

I personally take them every day, you can get them from most health stores, here is one I recommend:
BenHulme.com/omega3

4. Protein Shakes

Protein is an important component of every cell in the body. Your body uses protein to build and repair tissue. You also use protein to make enzymes, hormones, and other body chemicals. Protein is an important building block of bones, muscles, cartilage, skin and blood.

It's essential and a high protein diet will be directly beneficial to your success. This is especially true if we are working out, because protein will repair the damage we do to our muscles when we train which in turn will build them stronger and leaner so that we can adapt and transform.

The way we get protein into our body is important considering we need to keep our levels of protein high. You can of course eat meat and high-protein substitutes but it can get expensive and also time consuming to cook all the time.

I recommend you get yourself a high-quality protein shake as a supplement, it's what I do and have always done since I started. It's worth it, you will save so much time and money. It's not to replace natural protein sources, but to simply supplement your protein intake in a convenient manner.

You can get many different types of protein supplements but I recommend getting a low-carb version if your goal is to ultimately lose body fat.

For this reason, I recommend you go for a 'whey isolate' protein powder. It's low carb and high protein which is ideal for this nutrition plan.

You can choose any flavour you want but bear in mind that you may want to mix it with other things such as oats and fruit etc so choose flavours that would work for you. This is one of the places I recommend to buy your protein: **BenHulme.com/protein**

I often make my protein shakes with other ingredients in a Nutribullet so that they taste awesome. There is so much you can do with protein powder but the main advantage is the convenience factor.

The protein shakers you get from the shops are useful if you are out and about, but they aren't brilliant so I recommend a 'Nutribullet' for when you are at home: **BenHulme.com/ nutribullet**

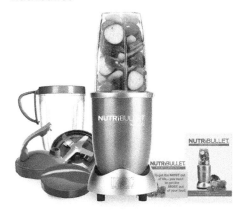

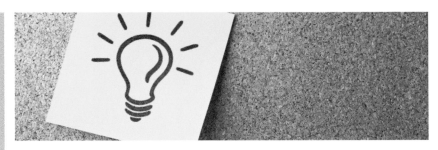

1. Portion size

Portion size is a key element to success with this nutrition plan. The idea is to be eating little and often, not a lot and often!

I used to load my plate up with as much food as I could and eat until I was completely full with every meal. This is because I used to eat food for pleasure rather than as a tool to transform my body.

This meant I was living my life in a calorie surplus and consuming more calories each day than I was burning and the result was evident, I put on weight.

Remember the laws of compound interest. Eating huge portions every now and then won't hurt but eating until you are full with every meal will compound into a negative effect on your body and your health.

My advice is to get a smaller plate and eat much slower. Having a big plate can be detrimental to your success with this because you can end up eating too much. If you have a smaller plate, you can't put so much food on it, therefore won't eat so much – problem solved!

You will need to eat often with this plan. That's the main 3 meals and then 3 snacks too. By eating on a smaller plate you can be sure that you won't be over eating and I recommend you only eat until you are 75% full. Never eat until you are 100% full, you just can't burn that off and you will be over eating which just isn't necessary.

You'll find that you will be eating a lot of food with this nutrition plan but it's food that your body needs. It's the food that we are designed to eat.

If you feel hungry you must eat more. You need to keep up your food intake to speed up your metabolism and don't forget to drink plenty of water.

2. Eat and cook as fresh as possible

The ultimate way to eat healthy is to cook with fresh ingredients.

As a personal trainer I hear a lot of excuses when it comes to eating and preparing food with fresh ingredients.

People say they don't have time to cook fresh food or that eating fresh food is too expensive.

They are valid reasons, but not necessarily true.

Good quality fresh food is now readily available and reasonably priced.
I personally find the pre-prepared, processed food is more expensive and obviously massively worse for you.

You can get fresh produce from supermarkets but also local farm stores which are often very cheap indeed. Just do some research into farm shops in your area.

When it comes to meat you get what you pay for. I would rather pay more money to get really good quality organic or free-range chicken and meat from the butchers than the cheap meat or processed meat from the supermarkets.

I guarantee you will feel so good eating fresh, healthy ingredients.

We all have busy lives and can of course make excuses regarding lack of time to eat healthy, but this type of cooking doesn't necessarily mean spending hours in the kitchen.

Here are some tips to help you:

1. When you're cooking your dinner it's a good idea to prepare a bit more so that you can have it as lunch (and snack 2) the next day. Not only does it save time but it will get you in the habit of eating healthy and fresh all day.

2. Prepare food for the week ahead if that will help you. Preparing the food on a Sunday for example means you can freeze and reheat as necessary during the week.

3. Eat veggies raw if you are in a rush. This way you have next to no preparation time and you get all the benefits from the nutrients without anything being lost in the cooking process.

4. Use the oven as much as possible. This means that while your food is cooking you can get on with other things without having to stand over a frying pan. It's super efficient and uses less oil in the cooking process so it's actually a super clean way to cook your food.

Important things to remember

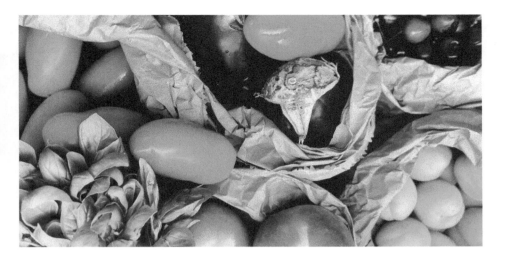

I believe that there are always solutions or excuses enabling us to eat fresh and healthy or not. That's why I've designed this plan to not only give you the understanding of how you can transform your body but also to give you the tools and knowledge to implement it.

I recommend that you buy meat from a butcher and fruit and vegetables from a greengrocers, if possible, that way like me you're also supporting local businesses.

I used to eat microwave meals for convenience but once I discovered how incredible I felt when eating fresh, I changed my diet permanently. You will too, I guarantee it.

Avoid processed food as much as possible. Processed food contains added sugar, salt and fats to preserve it for longer periods of time and to make the flavours more appealing.

This means that people tend to eat more than the recommended daily amount of sugar, salt and fat but more importantly these additional ingredients simply aren't healthy. Eat fresh food with lots of colour! Your plate shouldn't be beige, it needs to be colourful and as fresh as possible.

Make it happen and enjoy the results from your dedication. I recommend following this plan for at least 12 weeks and once you're satisfied with your progress, you can make small adjustments so that it's 100% sustainable for you **(whilst keeping to the guidelines)**.

THE BOOT CAMPER

Food you should be eating every day

1. Vegetables

Eating vegetables is important for a number of reasons. Vegetables provide nutrients such as potassium, dietary fibre, folic acid, vitamin A, and vitamin C; which are all vital for the health and maintenance of our bodies.

Eating a diet rich in vegetables as part of an overall healthy diet may also reduce the risk of some chronic heart diseases, heart attacks and strokes.

Within this plan you can eat any vegetables – except for refined, starchy carbs as mentioned in the next chapter **(except for your cheat meals)**. Simply aim for as much colour on your plate as possible and for the best nutritional value, choose a variety of vegetables. This will also keep your meals interesting and packed with flavour.

I recommend eating your vegetables either raw, grilled, roasted in the oven or steamed (which does the least amount of damage to nutrients during cooking, as boiling vegetables will result in a loss of nutrients in the cooking water).

Boiling is the next best thing and if that's how you like to cook your vegetables then that's fine and won't be a major issue.

Whether you like them or not, vegetables are good for you. They're an essential part of this plan and a huge part of your new healthy lifestyle.

2. Protein

Eating good quality protein is not only essential for this nutrition plan to work but it also has major benefits for weight loss and metabolic health and as we said earlier: we need protein to repair and sustain our development.

It's important to eat the right amount and the right kind of protein to receive all of the health benefits but also to assist with our body transformation.

So, first we need to understand the difference between 'good' protein and 'bad' protein.

Food you should be eating everyday

Proteins are found in both animal and vegetable sources. However, you'll find different varieties and different amounts of amino acids, which are the individual chemical units (building blocks) that contain the protein.

Good proteins, are those that provide all of the essential amino acids in a proportion needed by the human body. When looking for healthy protein meat sources, consider the following: chicken, turkey, lean beef, lamb, pork, fish and shellfish.

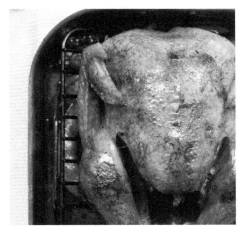

The general rule of thumb I use is that if it's processed or if it contains high saturated fat, then it's a bad protein.

Examples of bad meat proteins include, 'wafer thin' ham, sausages, burgers, fish cakes, fish fingers, bacon, ribs and all other fatty meats (combinations) are most certainly out of the question.

Start eating the best protein by making the right purchasing and preparation decisions:

• Read the packaging and choose lean cuts of meat where possible i.e. choose extra-lean or lean rather than regular ground beef.

• The type of meat i.e. opt for chicken breast with no skin instead of the fatty meat or 'drumsticks' and 'wings'.

• Buy good quality, free-range or organic meat. Cheap meat is pumped full of growth hormones and antibiotics, to extend the shelf life. I advise that you talk to your local butcher or the person working at the superstore behind the meat counter to see what they would recommend.

• Remove all excess fat before cooking.

• When cooking meat, drain the juices (contains a lot of fat) off while it's cooking.

As mentioned before, protein shakes are great. They're a cheaper option to get protein into your body without spending a fortune. They also don't take up a lot of time to prepare and can help with that sweet kick that you may crave. Remember that protein shakes are only a supplement and should never replace normal protein sources.

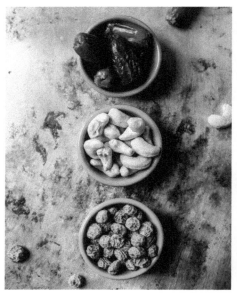

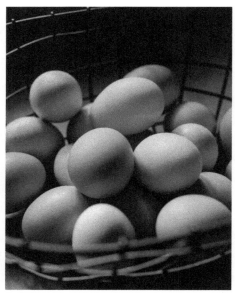

3. Nuts and seeds

Nuts and seeds provide a great natural source of nutrients including protein, fibres and essential fats, however should always be eaten in moderation.

I recommend only eating a small handful every other day or like me, on the days I workout. Opt for the plain rather than the sweetened or sugar-coated varieties.

4. Eggs

Eggs are rich in many nutrients, high in protein and easy to prepare. Personally I prefer to boil or scramble mine (no butter or milk) and on average will have 4 eggs a day but I would have 2 full eggs and 2 egg whites.

Egg whites contain the bulk of the egg's protein. The yolk is a major source of vitamins and minerals but also contains all of the fat. So again think carefully before eating too many yolks.

Foods to avoid with this plan

For the ultimate results and to achieve effective fat loss, I recommend that you completely avoid the list of foods below, as I did when transforming my body.

My advice is to stay as committed to this as you can, the stricter you are the faster you will see the results. If you don't buy these foods at all, then you can't give into temptation.

1. No more sugar

Let's start with the biggest problem. SUGAR!

Sugar provides absolutely no nutritional value. NOTHING. You simply don't need it. The problem is that we've all become addicted to refined sugars and therefore end up craving it.

2. Refined carbohydrates

Carbohydrates (carbs) form an essential part of a healthy balanced diet. Understanding the two types of carbs will help you achieve optimum results. Remember carbs are energy!

You might have heard the phrase: 'good carbs vs. bad carbs'? Both carbs are absorbed and processed differently and therefore have a different effect on our bodies. The 'good carbs' actively help to transform our bodies, whilst 'bad carbs' are not only detrimental to weight loss but also help to increase body fat.

Good carbs are known as unrefined carbs. These carbs are great sources of energy. Good carbs take much longer to be broken down and digested by our bodies, without having a negative impact on our blood-sugar levels.

Bad carbs are known as refined carbs. Bad carbs are quickly digested and cause a spike in blood-sugar levels. This simply means that if we don't burn off this energy, it is stored as fat.

The usual suspects for bad carbs are: Sugar, white potatoes, bread, pasta, white rice, potato chips/fries etc. I recommend you avoid these altogether except for your cheat meals where you can enjoy yourself a bit more.

Some examples of 'good carbs' that YOU SHOULD eat are: Porridge oats, couscous, quinoa, brown rice, bulgur wheat, whole-grain pasta, sweet potatoes etc.

These are the carbs that will dramatically improve your health and provide you with the necessary amounts of energy that is absorbed in a healthy way.

3. No more cheese

We don't need to say too much about cheese, other than it has a very high fat content and to obtain the ultimate results from this nutrition plan, all cheese except cottage cheese, should be avoided. You can of course include a small amount of cheese in your weekly cheat meal.

4. Choose your breads carefully

Typically, bread contains all sorts of additional ingredients such as sugar, oil, vinegar, preservatives and flour treatment agents that add no nutritional value to our diets. In fact, the gluten found in most bread can cause bloating.

If you must have bread, it's best to only have one slice of a freshly baked wholegrain loaf. I recommend that factory-baked loaves that are mass produced or pre-cut, should be avoided altogether.

5. Remove all sugary condiments & processed cooking sauces

We've all used some type of condiment, table sauce or cooking sauce to either provide a specific flavour, or, to enhance the flavour of a meal.

I, as much as anyone else, don't want to eat bland food, but condiments like tomato ketchup, BBQ sauce, salad dressings, mayonnaise and other pre-prepared cooking sauces that we harmlessly add to our food, are often full of sugars, fat, sodium and nasty preservatives; all of which cause weight gain.

Instead of condiments, I recommend adding fresh or dried herbs and spices to your meals. You can get an incredible flavour with these alone and they are readily available at most supermarkets. Remember to avoid sugary rubs though.

You can also replace salad dressing with extra virgin olive oil, some balsamic or white wine vinegar and lemon juice.

I love spicy food myself and for a bit more flavour every now and again, I'll add a small amount of hot sauce, for example Tabasco. I also use a little Worcestershire sauce and sometimes a little English mustard.

The hotter the sauce the better, as you get a lot of flavour without having to add too much sauce on your food. However, I fully appreciate that spicy food isn't for everyone!

Food to avoid with this plan

Like with everything, if you aren't sure what's in the product it's best to check the labels. As a general rule of thumb, if it contains a high amount of sugar or a list of unhealthy ingredients, it's best to completely avoid it.

If you can't eat food without ketchup then you are best to buy the reduced sugar and reduced salt versions. That will make a huge difference but in an ideal world, cut out the sugary condiments altogether.

Check out this awesome 100% healthy protein ketchup. I personally use it on a lot of my meals. There is literally nothing bad in it at all. The ingredients are totally on plan and it's a great substitute for regular table sauces.

You can get 20% off by using promo code: 'TheBootCamper' at
www.In-The-Buff.uk

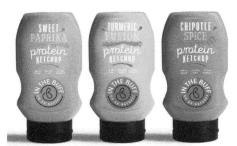

6. Cooking oils

Most, if not all of the food recommended in this nutrition plan can be cooked using either the oven or a grill as a substitute to frying. By using alternative cooking methods, you'll easily be able to avoid cooking with unhealthy cooking oils, including vegetable and olive oil.

Should you wish to fry any foods I recommend that you use a good quality non-stick frying pan for 'dry frying' OR add a little water or no more than a teaspoon of coconut oil.

Why you shouldn't cook with olive oil?

Olive oil changes its molecular properties when it's cooked and our bodies struggle to break it down. You can however use raw olive oil as a dressing on salads, it's really good for you.

If you have to fry with oil, then I would recommend using coconut oil only. There are arguments for and against the use of coconut oil for frying food, personally I use it, but you can make your own decision on this.

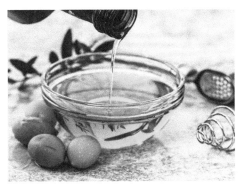

7. Cut out the salt

The majority of the salt we consume every day is hidden in the foods we eat, therefore cutting out salt is not just as simple as removing it from your dining or kitchen table.

The best bet is to avoid all processed foods and microwave meals which contain high amounts of salt.

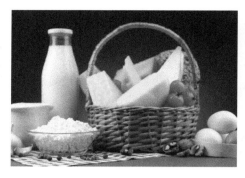

8. Cut down on dairy

For this nutrition plan to work effectively, it's best to avoid dairy (butter, milk or cheese) as much as possible and switch to an alternative such as unsweetened almond milk.

It was hard for me at first to switch from white to black coffee however the health benefits of removing dairy for me, made it worth it. If you have to have milk in your tea or coffee, then a little won't be the end of the world but try to avoid it where you can.

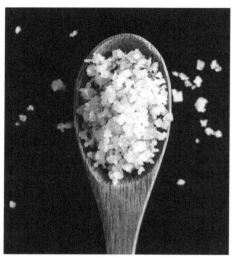

But why do we cut out salt?

The amount of salt we eat, directly impacts our blood pressure. Salt makes your body hold onto water and if you eat too much salt, the extra water stored raises your blood pressure.

It's a well-known fact that the higher your blood pressure, the greater the strain on your heart, kidneys, arteries and brain, which can lead to a heart attack, stroke, dementia and kidney disease.

It's recommended that you should take a supplement to be sure you get your calcium source if you are not getting it from dairy, almond milk, soya milk or oat milk each day. You can get calcium as a supplement with many good quality multivitamins.

Food to avoid with this plan

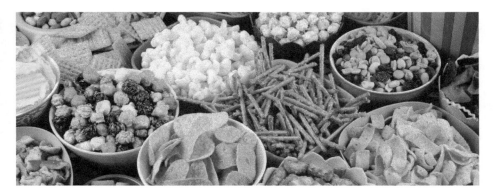

9. Avoiding treats, bad snacks and overcoming cravings

We all know this is a necessary evil. It's hard to accept but the naughty treats have to stop!

Earn your cheat meal. Earn your treat. It'll be worth it I promise. But if you really are desperate, then one or two squares of 80–90% cocoa chocolate will be enough to satisfy a sweet tooth every now and again.

However, for this nutrition plan to successfully work, you must eat little and often but this means eating the right snacks and avoiding the bad ones.

No excuses. Reread the mindset section within this book and commit to this. Remember everything you eat either takes you towards your goals or away from them.

I'm sure it's not news to you that chocolate, sweets, biscuits, crisps/chips, puddings or desserts and other sweet treats will prevent you from seeing the success you desire. Not only that but it will also undo any of your hard work and any effort you've made towards becoming the best version of yourself.

Luckily there are other options to help with sugar cravings.

I find a good quality herbal tea, a protein shake or even chewing a piece of gum, relieves cravings. Over time your cravings will subside as you lose the 'addiction' to sugary foods. I promise, it gets easier.

It's the small sacrifices that you make now that will force your body to adapt and that will get you to where you want to be in the future. Trust me, it might be hard at first, but it's so very worth it.

THE BOOT CAMPER

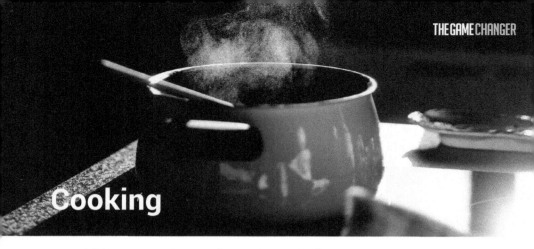

Cooking

In addition to understanding what foods to eat and why, food preparation and cooking is super important to the success of your body transformation. If you don't cook for yourself, I recommend that you read this section to the person who does the cooking at home, to ensure you stay on plan.

In my opinion, for long-term commitment to this plan and to sustainably transform your body; food preparation and cooking needs to be relatively quick and easy.

Complex recipes that are almost always time consuming are a chore and a deterrent and because of this, most diet plans become unsustainable. Remember, we aren't eating for pleasure, we are using food as a tool to achieve the desired results for our bodies.

The fundamentals:

• If you are new to cooking, my best advice is to be organised before you start cooking. Ensure that you've done all of the necessary food preparation to avoid overcooking or burning different parts of the meal.

• As we said before, avoid cooking with unhealthy cooking oils, including vegetable and olive oil.

• Always aim to oven bake, grill and roast instead of frying or deep-fat frying.

• Boil, steam, roast and use the microwave (although I try to avoid it) for cooking vegetables. I recommend steaming as it retains most of the nutrients.

• If you use other cooking appliances, like a slow cooker, be mindful of what you include with the food i.e. sauces, salt, sugars etc.

Cooking

No one likes boring food

Nutrition plans or healthy eating is often associated with boring or tasteless food, due to the perception of having fewer or limited options.

I want to tell you now; healthy food doesn't have to be boring at all. Nevertheless, there's a big difference between healthy food that's good for you and tastes great and unhealthy food that tastes great but is bad for you.

Cooking with natural ingredients like fresh herbs and spices, chili, lime or lemon juice, ginger, Thai mixes and Indian herb mixes can add a lot of flavour to any meal. In fact, chillies help to speed up your metabolism and burn fat faster so it's a highly recommended addition to your meals because you don't need that much to get a lot of flavour.

Healthy food can taste great and doesn't have to be boring despite what people say.

I don't like boring food, so I make sure that everything I cook is packed with flavour so that it never gets boring and is a sustainable solution for living a healthy lifestyle.

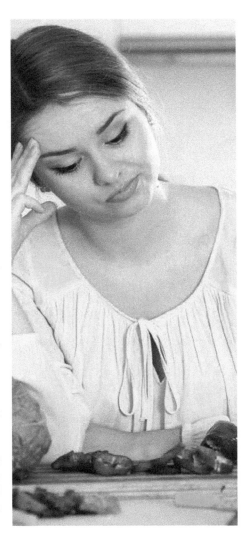

THE
BOOT
CAMPER

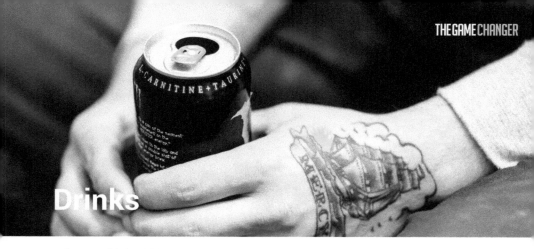

Drinks

What we drink will have a huge impact on our body transformation.

We've discussed why water is important under 'Essentials To Get You Started', which is worth revisiting again on page 40.

This section is however, all about the other drinks that you can or can't drink if you want to transform your body fast.

No more soft drinks or energy drinks

This first one might be hard for you. I struggled at first giving up the fizzy drinks (you know the usual suspects). However this was a real game changer for me.

Soft drinks and energy drinks contain carbonated water, sweeteners, flavourings, caffeine, preservatives, chemicals and 'e-numbers' that can be really harmful to our bodies.

Most importantly, these drinks contain a staggering amount of sugar. In fact, did you know some cans of fizzy drinks have up to 9.5 teaspoons or 33 grams of sugar? As we've said before, refined sugar provides absolutely no nutritional value and furthermore it can't be broken down by our bodies, so instead is stored as fat.

Remember we talked about compound interest? Let's do a few calculations...

2 cans a day = 730 cans per year and 6,935 teaspoons of sugar per year, just from those soft drinks.

4 cans a day = 1,460 cans per year and 13,870 teaspoons of sugar per year.

Just take a moment to think about what that's doing to your health and your body. Instead, switch to water! Once you see the results from eliminating sugary drinks you will love the new you, which makes it totally worth it.

I often cut some fruit like lemons and lime into my drinks to make it taste better, it also helps with your digestion.

Drinks

Milk

Milk is a controversial topic. But for this plan, milk is to be avoided wherever possible. If you need to have a dash of milk in your tea or coffee it won't hurt but if you do, then reach for skimmed milk only.

I personally drink unsweetened almond milk, instead of cow's milk. Almond milk is not to everyone's taste, however suitable substitutes are unsweetened soya milk, rice milk or oat milk.

At the end of the day, milk is designed to make a calf grow. The only benefit to milk is its calcium properties, which we need as children growing up. We now have access to other sources and supplements that provide us with the recommended amount of calcium.

It's recommended that you should take a supplement to be sure you get your calcium source if you are not getting it from almond milk, soya milk or oat milk etc each day. You can get calcium as a supplement with many good quality multivitamins.

Tea and Coffee

This is up to you. I know a lot of people can't function without a cup of tea or coffee. Personally I refuse to give up coffee. I love it and it's something that I am actually quite passionate about. I love nothing more than going for a coffee with friends and family in the morning.

As you might know, tea and coffee contain a high amount of caffeine, which can aid fat loss but can also reduce the amount of deep sleep necessary for fat loss.

Therefore it's recommended to stop drinking caffeine after 4pm. Green tea is a suitable alternative to tea or coffee.

It's full of antioxidants and nutrients that can improve brain function, encourage fat loss and lowers the risk of cancer. However green tea still contains caffeine.

Herbal and fruit teas are fantastic and can stop sugar cravings.

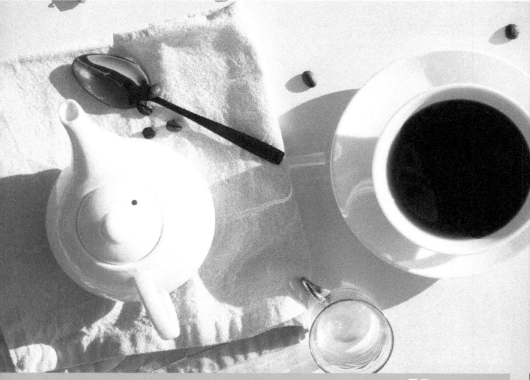

Drinks

Alcohol

People enjoy alcohol for different reasons, whether socially or as part of a meal. However the health implications of alcohol is thoroughly researched and documented in various studies around the world.

For the purpose of this plan, it is worth noting that alcohol slows down your metabolism. It can also negatively affect your sleep, your digestion and nutrient absorption.

A beer or glass of wine every now and again is generally fine, however to ensure that this nutrition plan is as effective as it could be and to achieve the ultimate body transformation, it's best to avoid alcohol as much as possible, even on a weekend when you might be more tempted.

It all comes down to how badly you are wanting to transform your body and how committed you want to be to that process.

The facts are simple, if you stop alcohol you will get better and faster results, if you don't then you will see slower results. The choice is yours entirely.

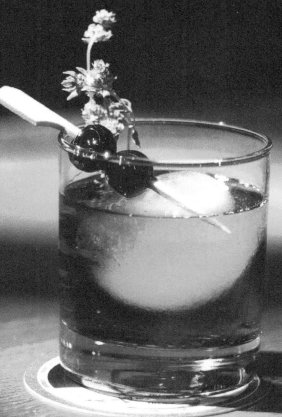

THE
BOOT
CAMPER

Get plenty of sleep

SLEEP is crucial.

To sustain a healthy lifestyle and to function at your best, you need 8 hours of sleep every night.

Sleep is important to our physical and mental health. During sleep our bodies repair and recover and this helps to ensure healthy brain function. An insufficient amount of sleep causes fatigue, can increase the risk of heart disease, diabetes and high blood pressure to name but a few.

If like me you're a light sleeper, try to develop a better bedtime routine. This will improve not only your quality of sleep but also ensure that you're getting enough sleep.

It is completely normal that you may feel a little tired during the first few days of this plan. That's because you are avoiding blood-sugar spikes (as we explained in this book already), which in turn means that your body is forced to trigger the energy from your fat reserves rather then directly from the sugary carbs it's currently used to.

Most importantly however, listen to your body whilst you adapt to this new way of life.

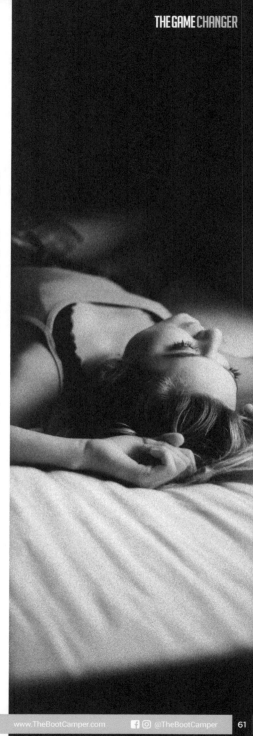

Cheat meals

YES! You can have cheat meals. This is the best thing about my nutrition plan, you get to reward yourself once a week, for all your hard work you've put in during that week.

A 'cheat meal' is a meal of your choice and it can be anything in moderation. Meaning you can have a social evening on a Friday or a Saturday night and perhaps even a glass of wine or a beer!

Personally I recommend that you have your cheat meal for lunch, that way your body has more time to burn it off throughout the day, however this is completely up to you.

Cheat meals are something I really do recommend and should be enjoyed but don't undo all your efforts of that week by having a full blown 10,000 calorie feast.

You are still on a body-transformation journey, so reward yourself and leverage this to get you through the next week.

The cheat meal will reset you for the week ahead, they're a very important part of this plan.

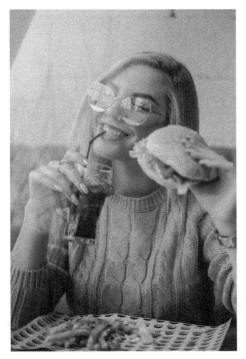

Unless you are a pro athlete or a pro bodybuilder, why be on a diet for your whole life? We have to enjoy the food we eat and when you get to your goals, maybe you could even switch to a cheat day and enjoy the food you like for that entire day each week.

You see, this doesn't have to be boring and a chore, this is a case of leveraging the nutrition plan to force your body to adapt and when you reach your goals, you can adjust accordingly.

If you have any questions about this you can always join our support community:
BenHulme.com/mentoring

Slip-ups and mistakes

Mistakes are going to happen, we're only human. Please don't be too hard on yourself. If you do make a mistake, regroup like I do and learn from it. Just keep asking yourself, is this going to take me towards or away from what I want to achieve?

We can all live a healthy lifestyle but there will always be that one event for example, a wedding that doesn't cater for your new lifestyle. We are normal people looking to transform our bodies, not pro athletes so don't let this stop you from enjoying your life.

Having one cheat meal on a weekend won't ruin the plan, it's all about compound interest and finding the balance for you.

Remember this is for a sustainable body transformation and a new healthy lifestyle, not a temporary quick fix!

On the next page you will find the 'Daily Plan Of Action' and the 'Daily Food Diary'. These are going to be very useful on your body-transformation journey.

You can download them for free at: **BenHulme.com/usefultools**

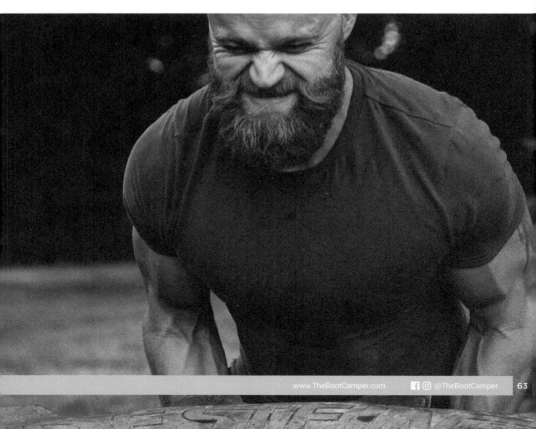

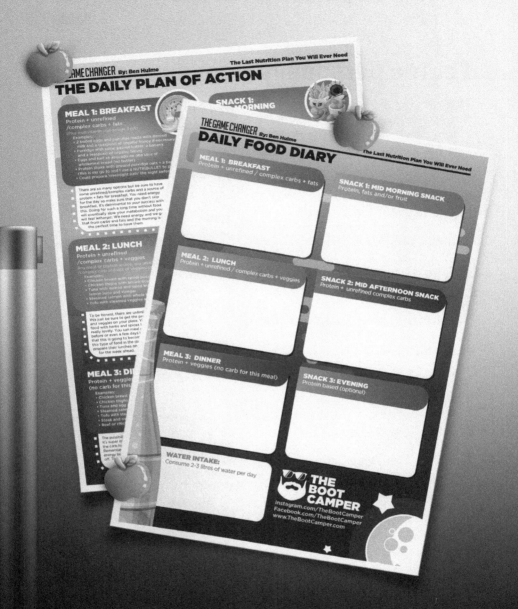

Download the DAILY ACTION PLAN and the DAILY FOOD DIARY with my compliments via my website.

You'll also discover FAQ's and much more via this link:
BenHulme.com/usefultools

Let me personally train you, virtually!

To really change the game I advise that you exercise and workout regularly. When combined with this nutrition plan you will be amazed at the results.

Many people hate the gym and having trained thousands of clients personally I have discovered many reasons why but that doesn't mean you need to neglect exercise. If you want your body to adapt, you will need to exercise to see the results you desire!

As you probably know, I run a successful boot camp in West Sussex, UK and I would love to see you there. Check it out at: **BootCampAtTulleys.com**

However, realistically it's not possible for everyone to get there so I have created an online workout platform to help people from all over the world.

It's called 'The Boot Camper' and it's an online video platform where I can personally train you from the comfort of your own home, in fact absolutely anywhere, anytime!

I have created a series of workout videos in the most amazing studio. Each movement has a full individual explainer video with 360 degree rotations so that you won't be left confused and can achieve the perfect form.

All you have to do is follow along as I take you through the progressive workouts as if I am there with you personally. This will force your body to adapt. You will tone muscle, get leaner, get stronger and ultimately drop that unwanted body fat.

It doesn't matter what your current fitness level is, even if you have never 'worked out' before because this is all about YOU vs YOU! By sticking to the plan you will progress week after week and you will be amazed at how your body will change.

The existing members of 'The Boot Camper' are seeing epic results and I want to personally invite you to join them as the next member of The Boot Camper.

You will never be alone or left in the dark because we also have a full help and support community where I'll be able to mentor you to success with your personal health and fitness journey.

I guarantee that this will work for you because I have done it myself. I would love for you to be the next success story!

I look forward to seeing you in the members area very soon.

Get started at **TheBootCamper.com**

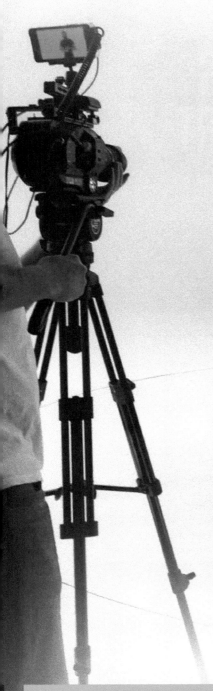
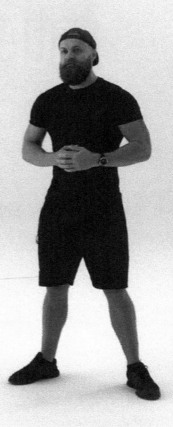

**Join The Boot Camper at
TheBootCamper.com**

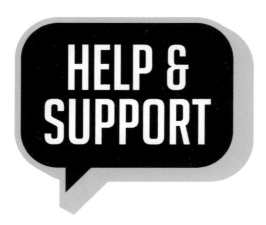

HELP & SUPPORT

If you would like further support, I recommend you join our growing community at **BenHulme.com/mentoring** where you will be able to meet like-minded people from all over the world who are on the same mission as you. You will become part of a group of people who want to help and support you as much as possible.

I am an active part of the community and post regular video updates and comments to help you on your journey. I also shoot live video Q&A sessions via our Facebook group to answer any questions.

If you haven't already, you can also check out my online workout platform.

Head to **TheBootCamper.com** so that you can run your own home-based boot camps with me as your personal trainer.

You can only go so far with diet alone, so if you really want the big results, join us as a member of The Boot Camper and I will show you how we workout at my boot camps.

Remember, we are designed to adapt, so force your body to adapt by fuelling yourself with what we are supposed to eat not what our society has created for us.

Listen, this will work for you, I guarantee it. It will be a game changer for you but remember, it's what you do when no one is watching that makes all the difference with this.

Commit to this and you will get results, don't and you won't. No one is going to do it for you. So let's make this happen together.

I can't wait to hear about your results with this.

I've got your back.

Ben Hulme
The Boot Camper
BenHulme.com
Instagram.com/benhulme
Facebook.com/benhulmeofficial